WHY PEOPLE FAIL IN FITNESS

The 17 Obstacles to
Success and How You
Can Overcome Them

ALEX ALVAREZ

To all the people struggling with failures in their life…

CONTENTS

INTRODUCTION

About me

My name is Alex. I have been working in the fitness industry since I was 16 years old. I have worked with 3 major kinds of people: The elite (semi-pro/ pro athlete), the injured/unwell (people dealing with health conditions such as arthritis or extreme obesity), and lastly, the normal average working person.

During many years of working very closely with such a variety of people, I have gained immense insight into their mind-set and habits. And through years of observation and experience I have come to understand what makes some people successful in fitness and health, while others remain frustrated and disappointed! This is essentially what I now do for a living; I coach people on their mind-set and habits so that they can then transform their bodies and become the fittest version of themselves.

Why I wrote the book

I wrote this book because I feel extremely frustrated at the fact that although there are so many fitness trainers, fitness articles, documentaries, apps, websites, social media influencers etc., out there, the vast majority of people are still completely lost and seem to have no clue what they're doing. Or worse, they really think they know a lot about what they are doing but are deluded and deep down are actually not happy with their progress at all.

Firstly, all this information out there can be really confusing for anyone that is not an expert. How is the average person supposed to know if the 'Keto Diet' or 'A Carb Cycling Diet' is best for them? Or supposed to know whether they should be doing 'Fasted HIIT' or standard steady state cardio?

Secondly, if you do happen to get the right info from a good source, most people still don't seem to know what to do with it. They don't know how to put it into action, practically, and as part of their daily life.

My goal was to write a book that is easy to understand for 'non-specialists', but still loaded with the useful things that actually matter and that makes it easy for normal people to TAKE ACTION from day 1!

Fit vs Unfit

Throughout this book, I use the terms 'Fit' and 'Unfit'. I am not talking about a person's actual fitness levels at all and not trying to create any form of negative labelling.

I am referring to the mind-set, beliefs & habits of a fit person vs an unfit person.

In each chapter I go through one of these mind-sets, beliefs or habits, and using common day to day examples, I show you how to be free from their grasp. If you follow the steps that I have laid out for you in each chapter, I guarantee that you will undergo a huge mental and physical transformation!

To Your Success!

Alex

A small note

Throughout this book I use some informal language, unorthodox grammar and casual (deliberate) spelling errors. This is simply because this is how I speak in 'real life' so will not pretend to be some Cambridge literature writer when I'm clearly not one. Now that we've cleared that up. Enjoy! :)

1. WE WANT IT ALL SO FAST; EXPECTATIONS AND SOCIAL MEDIA

It is human nature for us to compare ourselves with others. Whether in terms of income, looks, character, lifestyle etc. It's something we all instinctively do even if we try not to or claim we don't do. This would not be such a problem if we lived in a tiny remote village somewhere and we could only compare ourselves with those around us. But thanks to the media/social media we are now able to watch and observe the lives of the majority of the world. This means we, consciously or not, are comparing ourselves against the most successful, good looking and popular people in the world! It's not very fair for us to do that to ourselves is it?

The problem with social media is that what everyone presents is the best/perfect version of themselves.

You see:

- Their highlight reel; their best bits.

- Them become an overnight millionaire.

- Them drop 15% body fat in 90 days.

- Them at a luxury holiday with a gorgeous companion by their side.

These repetitive marketing messages have distorted our sense of what it really takes to succeed.

What you do not see:

- The countless hardships and failures the entrepreneur made when she was struggling hard to get her fashion e-commerce business off the ground.

- The amount of years Derrick spent yoyo dieting before finally adjusting his lifestyle and developing the mind-set where he could finally lose 10kg of fat in 90days.

- You do not see that actually all these jaw dropping holidays the 'influencer' takes was from years of building up a successful social media platform and a strong network. That he personally gets invited by VIPs to luxury locations.

6

1. Write down an example where you have been expecting results much faster than realistically possible, because of media/social media's influence on you.

2. You must remind yourself of these facts every time you consume media/social media! Otherwise you can get sucked in and develop a very unrealistic expectation of yourself which does you more harm than good. Use it as inspiration or education but never comparison.

As the famous quote says 'Comparison is the thief of joy' Theodore Roosevelt.

2. YOU'RE A SUCKER FOR A TREND!

If you've been in the game as long as I have you see trend after trend come and go; now it is important to note that I'm not saying all trends are fads. The problem is when you get sucked into the new craze, then jump to the next thing just as quickly as you jumped on the first.

- Years ago low fat diets were the thing, then came the Paleo Diet, now the Keto Diet, then Intermittent Fasting, Carb Cycling, rise of the Vegans, raw food Nazis. These trends go out of fashion then come back in again.

- Same applies to HIIT Classes, then Crossfit, Barry's Bootcamp, F45, LISS etc.

They are all TOOLS to get you to eat and exercise well. There are pros & cons of each, some may just be better suited to your character than others.

It's all about understanding the fundamentals, sticking to it and not jumping ship as soon as another trend pops up!

Fundamentals:

1. If you want to lose weight/fat then you NEED to eat less than you are burning.

2. Use any eating and exercise style to make this possible.

3. Do it CONSISTENTLY.

In Chapters 6 and 9, I'll go into more details on these fundamentals.

I encourage you all to experiment with a variety of training methods to see which one you enjoy the most and can see yourself remaining consistent with. I also recommend you try a variety of food plans to see which one suits your character the best, which one you enjoy the most and find the least restrictive.

BUT NEVER ignore the fundamentals!

Action Steps

1. Write down a time in your life where you were a sucker for a fad? What was it?

2. Did you find yourself changing from one fad to another and never really noticed a positive difference in the long term?

Before you continue:

Did you actually do the action steps? If your answer to this is "NO," then please do not continue until you have taken the few minutes necessary to do so.

3. NOT KNOWING YOUR 'WHY'?

When it comes to dropping body fat, gaining muscle, being healthy. Most people just 'kinda sorta' want it. But they don't *really* want it! Having an unclear and vague mindset will literally give you *no fuel* or power to follow through with the steps it takes you to get you to your dream version of yourself.

To really achieve something, you have to be committed to it. For you to be committed you need to:

1. Know **why** you want it.

2. Feel as though you **cannot bear to remain** another day as you currently are.

Everyone knows that setting goals brings what we want to achieve into clear focus and if we map out exactly how to get there then it makes it even more effective. But if you want to make your goal setting 10x more powerful you need to know WHY you are doing something and use 'Pain' as a motivation. We're not talking actual physical pain but more so from the disappointment of letting yourself down or the pain of having low self-esteem. I'll explain this a bit more on the next page.

Here's a quick one I love that shows this point wonderfully:

There are two 100m high buildings, 15m apart. Connecting both roofs I have put down a plank of wood just wide enough for you to walk across so you can go from one side to the other, but of course the risk of falling is high!

If I ask you would you walk across to the other side for £20? You would undoubtedly say no!

What if it was for £1,000? Hmm, I'm sure you would still say no!

BUT what if it was to save the life of your daughter, your niece, your nephew, your mother? Now, the answer I'm sure will be Yes!

So you see, *the situation has not changed*. All that has changed is your WHY.

When you want to achieve something; especially if it's something big or challenging, knowing your WHY & using pain is key! (In this case the pain of losing a loved one).

When I ask people *'Why do you want to achieve these goals?'*

Most people will say but I know why I want it *'I just want to get fit'*

This is the superficial answer

- Beyond that I ask my clients *'why do you want to get fit?'*

- They may say *'so I look good'*

- Then I say *'why do you want to look good?'*

In which we finally get to the real point! *'I hate feeling overweight and uncomfortable in my clothes/ naked and I want to feel good!'*

Which as you can clearly see has a lot more power to fuel motivation than just saying 'I want to get fit'.

Common Scenario

Imagine you've had a long day at work; you come home exhausted and need some energy. In that moment you are craving something very calorific because that's what your habit has been to do. You're trying to make better decisions so you think about your motivation (*why you want It*). If your motivation is '*I want to get fit*' it's so weak that you will most likely give in and just eat something very calorific. BUT, if your motivation is something powerful that involves PAIN such as '*I can't bear to feel so unfit that I can't even walk up the stairs without getting out of breath*'. Then you are much more likely to make your goals become your reality.

Most 'Fit' people know their WHY and this why they have the motivation to get the hard work done day in/day out!

Action Steps

1. Write down **what you want for yourself** - your new standard?

   I want to...e.g. Lose 10% body fat, improve strength etc by the time I hit my 35th Birthday or for my wedding, etc.

2. **WHY do you want it?** You need to find your pain point and why you can't bear to stay that way anymore.

   Because... Is it just to have less fat on your body? Or is it because the way you would FEEL if you freed yourself of those unwanted pounds, giving yourself more energy and vitality, making yourself more attractive to others, boosting confidence and self-esteem, feeling healthier and more physically able to perform day to day tasks with ease?

   What will it cost you if you don't change NOW?

Over the next two, three or five years, what is it going to cost to your health and physical well-being?

What is it going to cost you in terms of your self-image? What will it cost you in your relationships with people you care about the most (your partner or kids)?

3. You need to **make a plan to achieve it?**

    In order to fulfill my goal, I will…. e.g. Do 3 gym sessions per week (Mon, Weds, Friday 12noon), Log all my food in Myfitnesspal, Contact a trainer to help me, go to body pump classes, etc.

4. You need to constantly focus on **how good you will feel/do feel** for executing your plan.

    I will gain new physical vitality and health, I'll be more attractive to others, I'll feel more confident, I'll develop my willpower which I can use in other areas of my life etc.

5. **Every day**, read over these!

- Focus on the pain of the past.

- And focus on the joy you feel for working towards your dream.

- Make it part of your morning ritual to read over these, or save it as a screen saver on your phone. It needs to constantly be on your mind.

If you follow the above not only will you be clear on how to achieve your goals but you will also have that motivational fuel to make sure you follow through with the steps that get you there!

4. YOU DON'T TRACK YOUR PROGRESS!

'Unfit' people do not use any type of system to track their progress. They have a mind-set that they are better off following their 'gut instinct or listening to how their body feels' and expecting that it will deliver them favorable results. This is a hopeful and slightly naïve way of thinking at best.

The reality is you do not know your body anywhere near as much as you think you do. 'You're telling me your body has told you to eat high calorie/ poor quality food in excessive amounts that it needs to get stored as this extra fat all over your body?'

1. The first step towards change is **simply being aware of what you are currently doing;** this is where a system to measure your progress comes in. Now it doesn't need to be complicated but it needs to at the very least show you exactly what you are doing well and where there is room for improvement.

It could be:

System to track food

- Food Diary

- Fitness App like Myfitnesspal

- Photos of each Meal

Whatever it is, just trying to remember off the top of your head is not good enough.

In addition to it showing you the full effects of your actions, it will also keep you accountable and get you thinking twice about eating any crap because you will have to see yourself writing it down ☺

System to track training progress

If you're into strength training, then track weights, reps and sets.

  o Use apps like JeFit or even excel.

If you're into cardio, then track distance/ time/speed.

  o Maybe get a Fitness Watch with HR & GPS

This will stop you doing the same workout over and over again with no progress or results.

Everything nowadays involves measurables. Could you imagine going to work and then not checking how much you get paid at the end of the month? Or imagine if your boss would let you just turn up without having any tasks for you to do and never reviewed your progress as time goes on. How likely would that be? Or imagine if your kids go to a school where there was no work being marked, no progress reports and no grades being given. Would you let your kids go to such a school?

You get the idea. Using a system will always lead to faster and better results than without it. Otherwise you may aimlessly pass the time with no progress and never know why. Or you might even improve but have no idea how or why. Then when you hit a plateau (everyone does) you will have no idea how to overcome it.

For the record if your goal is simply to move and enjoy exercise that is fine but if you are disappointed with your progress, using a system to measure things is one of the first things you should do.

Action Steps

1. Choose a system that you think may work best for you.

2. Begin recording for a whole week and spend 10 minutes at the end of the week to evaluate how it's all gone. You will immediately see where you did some things well and where you may have room for improvement.

3. Make 1 or 2 small and achievable targets for the following week. Then evaluate progress at the end of the week.

Each week will be different. Some will be better than others. The only real mistake you can make here is giving up and going back to immeasurable action. My tip is that you make the targets for each week mega realistic so that you are not over-reaching and potentially setting yourself up for failure. Failure can be tricky for motivation.

5. YOU GO TOO EXTREME AND THEN CAN'T KEEP IT UP!

I get it... you want results fast. So you do something extreme like:

- Only eating apples and eggs for 1 week, Or

- Only drinking 'cleanse juices' and not eating solid food etc.

- Or you have a week off work so you train 7 days in a row after literally not having done anything for a year.

Which may result in you losing a large amount of weight in a short amount of time...BUT...

So what's the problem?

1. What you are losing **may not be quality fat tissue** and so even if you do lose 'weight' you may not get the toned look you desire because you have also lost shit loads of muscle in the process. ☹

2. You may pick up an **injury or get unwell.**

3. A bigger and much more important point that I want to emphasize is that something so extreme is **NOT SUSTAINABLE!**

What happens when your 7-day madness is over? You go back to eating the same foods and adopting the same habits as before. What happens when you have to go back to work and family? When will you fit in these 7 sessions per week? The answer: you won't fit in any.

Anyone that has ever done one of these extreme things ends up putting on the same amount of weight or more than they initially started with. **This cycle literally ends up going on for years of people's lives.**

When you ask such a person how the extreme diet is working for them, they often claim it's amazing, WHEN they follow it properly. BUT that's the fundamental point! It is almost impossible to follow for any longer than a few weeks max! It's not sustainable OR realistic OR normal!

Instead, we need to address the root cause of why they got fat in the first place; Habits and Lifestyle!!

A few simple things to look into first:

- How much are you walking?

- Do you go to the gym or not? How often?

- What are your eating habits like? (as mentioned above, a food diary or food diary app can help a lot here)

  1. How many meals do you eat per day?

  2. How many servings of protein?

  3. How many servings of veg?

  4. How much dessert do you have?

  5. How much alcohol do you drink per week?

This will all serve as your baseline of what you do if you answer all the above honestly.

Next step: how can you start integrating some better habits into your current life?

- 'Okay so my work is normally quiet around lunch. Are there any gyms near me? Yes? 2 minutes walk perfect? What classes do they have that I might like or is there a trainer that can help me? Yes there is. Great. I will go there 2 times per week because that is realistic for me at the moment.'

- 'I'm normally eating croissants for breakfast every day, can I eat something else that I also like instead that is better for me? Yes, Pret has a tasty porridge with berries. Great! I'll do that.'

If you have the above mindset and you make 1 small improvement per week CONSISTENTLY over the course of a year, you will be in the best shape you have ever been in. AND you will be able to keep it up forever because you are being realistic and integrating healthy choices into your EXISTING life, rather than simply trying to just jump into the lifestyle of a fitness model overnight!

Action Steps

1. Write down the answers to the questions on page 27 about activity, diet and lifestyle.

2. Write down 2 habits you can begin to integrate into your current lifestyle starting from next week!

3. Re-evaluate this every few weeks and see if you can integrate another 2 habits.

6. EAT NOURISHING FOOD FIRST; BEFORE DROPPING CALORIES!

'Unfit' people go wrong in the following way:

Firstly, the reason they have become fat is because they are eating too many calories compared to what they are burning. They are eating too many calories because their body is craving good nutrition. If they are giving it sub-par nutrition, then their body will crave a larger quantity of food to be satisfied and even then, they will never quite feel truly satisfied; they simply feel stuffed but never properly satisfied.

So for most people when the goal is fat loss, they immediately START by trying to eat less. This goes okay for a day or 2 and yes they will lose weight BUT then the cravings kick in! They feel they are starving because they haven't worked on giving their body quality nutrients first!

We're talking the right amounts of:

- Protein (amino acids), Fats (good quality fatty acids), Carbs (clean ingredients)
- Vitamins
- Minerals ⎱ A large amount of these mainly come from plants
- Anti-oxidants

1. For ALL of my clients I get them to record a food diary so we can both see what they are and are not having.

2. Then I immediately get them working on getting more of the above quality nutrients, prioritising protein & green vegetables first! This is because our western diet is already high in carbs and fats so here we focus our attention on the nutrients that we are most lacking in! (protein, vitamins, minerals & anti-oxidants)

We Start with:

Getting in more **Protein**, but WHY?

- Very filling and tasty.

- 30% is burned, simply in the process of breaking it down.

- Eating more of it improves lean muscle (with the right training); which means in-creased metabolism.

- Also boosts immune system.

Examples: Any meat, fish, some seafood, low-fat yoghurt

Getting in more **Vegetables**, but WHY?

- Very filling and can be tasty.

- Packed with vitamins & minerals that boost energy, optimize hormones and are anti-cancer/anti-aging.

- Some vegetables also burn calories just to break them down.

Examples: Any green veg e.g. kale, spinach, broccoli

If you eat enough of the above you will be so nutri-tionally satisfied that you will feel so strong, ener-getic, healthy and your cravings will be massively reduced! Making it easier for you to lose fat.

ONLY once the good nutrients have been successfully

introduced into your daily eating, does it finally become time

to start finding creative ways to **drop calories.**

How much is enough?

A good Initial daily target is:

For Men - 140-160g Protein and 300-400g Veg.
For Women - 80-100g Protein and 200-300g Veg.

What about the other nutrients like carbs & fats? Are they not important?

Once again as mentioned earlier, since our diets are already so high in carbs and fats, at this stage focusing on getting enough protein and veg is our number one thing to focus on. Once this has been mastered, we can reduce portions of carbs and fats in order to drop calories.

1. Write down all the protein sources that you really enjoy eating. (USE GOOGLE for top sources ☺)

2. Write down all the vegetables that you really enjoy eating. We're talking green or coloured veg here, not potatoes etc.

3. On your next food shop, load up your basket with these things in addition to your normal shopping.

4. When deciding what to eat, select 1 protein that you love and 1 veggie that you love first, then build the meal around that!

7. SWITCHING THINGS UP TOO MUCH.

Most 'unfit' people are impatient and have a very unrealistic idea of how long it takes to get the results they expect. (If you've read chapter 1 you know that social media may be the one to blame). So, if after a few weeks, or even a few days in some cases of following an exercise programme or eating regime, they feel like it's not working as fast as they expect, they end up making drastic changes, instead of just small adjustments.

The following scenarios help explain why this is a problem.

Let's say Becky's goal is to drop body fat.

Becky starts eating in a way that burns more calories than she is taking in (calorie deficit). Week 1 she loses 1 kg so is really happy. Week 2 she loses 0.5kg and still feels okay but is slightly disappointed. Week 3 she loses no weight and decides that the diet is rubbish and doesn't work for her so binges for a day or two. Once the binge is over, starting at square one again, she decides to start a different diet.

- Instead, all that she needed to do was make a *small tweak* such as reducing her serving of bread for dinner each night or halving the amount of glasses of wine she has in a week. This would have been enough to keep her progressing for another week or 2.

Sound like someone familiar?

Another example is the guy that goes to the gym 3 days per week and is trying to build muscle; mainly his chest and arms. He's been following a program for 8 weeks but hasn't increased the weights or reps or sets. He noticed progress in the first 2 weeks but then nothing since. He read somewhere that you should always switch up your training, so, he completely changed his routine, once again noticing a small change for the first 2 weeks but then nothing after. He's been doing this for 2 years and not progressing much.

- All he needed to do was after 2 weeks in, was increase the weight by 2.5kg or add 2 reps or an extra set on each exercise and that would be enough to stimulate new growth! Then repeat the same again after another 2-4 weeks.

38

You MUST decide to have a mind-set that you are going to stick to a plan for the long term! If after a few weeks of following something religiously there is no progress or not as much progress as before, then make one small change.

- It could be changing what you have for breakfast each day.

- Or slightly increasing the weights on an exercise.

- Or increasing the distance of your run by 500m.

BUT whatever you do, do not change the whole diet or exercise programme! Believe me you will end up doing this for the rest of your life and end up believing that no programme works. It's not the programme that doesn't work it's YOU!

The name of the game here is:

1. Follow a system.

2. Evaluate your progress.

3. Make a small adjustment.

4. Improve.

1. Write down an example of a time when you kept switching things up too much? Was it effective? Where did it get you?

2. Using the above example how could you have made a minor adjustment that may have been more effective instead?

8. HOW LACK OF SLEEP DESTROYS OUR ABILITY TO LOSE FAT.

Okay you know sleep is 'important' but **how exactly** does it affect your ability to lose fat? Sleeping less than you need over a few days has a huge ripple effect on a variety of different things that influence fat loss:

1. **Kills Your Willpower** - We only have a certain amount of mental energy to fuel us through the day. It gets us to focus on the various tasks we encounter during the day. From work stressors, to driving, to worrying about what's for dinner, problems with your wife/ husband etc. We all know what it's like when we've used up this daily mental energy and our brain feels fried. When you are tired and lacking in sleep this only gets worse and you have even less mental energy (willpower). By the time you get home and are drained the last thing you are thinking is '*let me be super disciplined about my diet*' or '*I'm so exhausted why don't I just work out?*'

It just doesn't happen that you think this way and end up slacking off and doing the 'easiest option' even if it's not the best for you.

2. **Slows down metabolism** – Your body dooen't function at its full capacity while its sleep deprived. Any basic function such as digestion, energy production, hormone secretion are all working in a sub-optimal way which results in more fat storage in and around the body.

3. **Our training is less productive and effective** – When sleep deprived we can't train as hard or to the same quality so we burn less calories & stimulate the muscles less.

4. **Increased risk of injury** – Many research papers document the increased risk of injury from lack of sleep. This means having to take more time off training; once again affecting fat loss.

5. **Increased appetite** – Because of this lack of energy, from being under recovered and our body processes not producing energy optimally any more, we start to crave energy from other areas. Yup, you guessed it. Food! We become hungrier than normal and start to have all these wild cravings that we feel we must satisfy ☺

How much should I sleep?

It really depends on age, physical activity, stress but I'd say ideal is 7-8 hours for most people and you shouldn't be getting any less than 6-7 for more than 2 nights in a row.

Action Steps

Tips to fall asleep like a champ!

1. Make sure your bedroom is only for 2 things:
One is sleep and the other is ;)

Create an environment where your body starts to only associate your bedroom with sleep.

- This means No TV or Devices

- Keep these things for the living room.

2. Avoid artificial lights during hours of no natural sunlight!

Lol. But how am I supposed to function around my house during winter months when it gets dark at 4pm?

Answer: Use Blue light blocking glasses

How it works (in simple language)

When it's daylight we produce alertness/action hormones that get us ready to handle the day.

When it's dark, we produce repair/recovery hormones.

In this context at least, our bodies cannot tell the difference between artificial light (devices etc) and natural light. So if you're trying to sleep and exposing yourself to loads of artificial light right before bed, it's no wonder you are finding it hard to sleep deeply and peacefully.

How do the glasses work?

They block the blue light (which is the part of the light spectrum that influences these hormones the most). Even most mobile phones nowadays have a blue-light blocking feature where the screen is yellow after a certain time to help with this problem.

https://www.amazon.co.uk/Blue-Light-Blocking-Glasses-Artificial/dp/B0784MVXG2/ref=sr_1_7_a_it?ie=UTF8&qid=1535573887&sr=8-7&keywords=blue+light+blocking+glasses

9. YOUR TRAINING IS ALL WRONG; YOU STILL KEEP DOING 'CARDIO' FOR FAT LOSS!

When 'unfit' people want to lose weight they immediately think that they need to do 'cardio'. Now the reason they think this is because they think cardio burns the most calories.

- They may not be wrong that a 60 min run could burn 800kcals compared with a weight session that might burn just 600kcals.

Before we go further, let's break down what cardio actually means in simple language:

All it means is when your heart rate is working above a certain level for an extended period of time. That's it! This means that anything can be cardio providing we keep working our heart at a certain intensity (110-190 beats per min):

- It could be weight training, cycling, boxing, a bodyweight circuit, anything.

- It all depends how we arrange things to keep our heart rate up.

- In fact, in my experience you can arrange full body movements like squats and clean & press to give you an even greater calorie burn than running.

Weight training vs conventional cardio for fat loss:

'Conventional cardio' such as running:

- Only burns calories DURING the session (and maybe a bit after).

- Does nothing to increase the amount of calories you burn during the remaining 23 hours of the day.

Weight Training on the other hand (providing you are doing it in a particular way) does the following:

- Burns calories DURING the session.

- Builds strength and improves posture.

- MOST importantly though, it increases muscle which is very useful because the more muscle you have on you, the more you burn during the remaining 23 hours of the day (even when you sleep).

- It also makes your body look nice and toned.

For the record, I have nothing against conventional cardio and I'm a big fan of people doing it if they enjoy it. I'm simply saying it's not the most effective tool for fat loss.

An example of how little muscle is a problem.

An 80kg man with 30% body fat might need to eat as low as 1600-1800 calories to lose weight. Whereas, here I am at 80kg, needing to eat at least 2800 just to maintain weight. This is because I happen to have a few kilos more muscle than your average man. You might say "oh but you're a trainer Alex you train all day!" I'm ONLY training 3 days per week! But my sessions are intense and full body in nature!

Action Steps

So what might a weight training session for fat loss look like?

- Firstly, I recommend you get a coach or trainer to go through this with you so your form and everything is okay and to ensure that the exercises are tailored to giving you the physique you want.

- Here's an example for a semi-athletic Male in his mid-30s

  - ☐ 5 sets of (Squats 10 reps immediately into Banded Pull-ups 10 reps, rest 90 sec)

  - ☐ Then, 4 sets of (Bench press 10 reps immediately into Romanian deadlifts 10 reps, rest 90 sec)

  - ☐ Then 3 sets of (Military press 10 reps immediately into walking lunges 20m, rest 90 sec)

Something along the lines of that, 3 days per week is ideal!

10. SOMETIMES, THE LITTLE THINGS, CAN BECOME REALLY BIG THINGS, OVER TIME.

Your biggest challenge isn't that you've been deliberately making bad choices. Your biggest challenge is that you've been sleepwalking through your choices. That's the scary thing, half the time you're not even aware you're making them!

Nobody *intends* to become obese, get a divorce or become broke. Often, those consequences are a result of a series of small, poor choices over time.

Here's a scenario:

You are trying to lose body fat. What if I told you all you need to do is eat **200** calories less per day (than what you need for maintenance). You would laugh and say 'that's nothing!' or 'that's easy!' All that is 2 less cans of Coke or 3 less biscuits, etc.

It's an easy adjustment to make but in **1 week** that's **1400** calories less.

In **4 weeks** that's **1.6lb** of fat loss (3500 calories in 1 lb of fat)

In **1 year** that's **20.8lbs** of fat loss

You might say it's not much but that's the easiest 10kgs you've lost in your life! And it's all from:

Small Smart Choices + Consistency + Time = Big Difference

And it can work in reverse too! Just eating 200 calories extra per day can result in 10kg of extra fat on your body in 1 year; without even noticing, it just happens!

Action Steps

1. Write down a few small, seemingly insignificant actions/habits that may be stopping you from losing weight? E.g.

- Getting a cappuccino every morning

- Drinking a can of coke everyday

- Always using transport or lifts, barely any walking

- Been squatting the same weight for the last year

11. REPLACING BAD HABITS WITH GOOD ONES.

One of the major keys to long term change is understanding the power of habits!

Unfit people: Go wrong because they simply try to remove a bad habit without replacing the bad habit with a better one. An example is a person that suddenly decides not to eat anything sweet. They manage this for a few days or so but after a while they feel this void so end up entertaining another bad habit such as randomly deciding they will start eating more cheese or drinking more alcohol than normal.

This is because it simply feels weird when a habit is completely removed and not replaced by something else, our very nature wants to replace a removed habit with another habit in its place.

Fit people: They understand this fact so they replace bad habits with better ones. Such as: instead of ordering a 3000kcal Pizza from Firezza or Papa Johns, they will buy a frozen pizza from Waitrose that is only 700kcals!

The unfit people might argue: *'but surely you should be removing all bad habits? Not just replacing them with slightly less bad ones!'*

This is true, the long term game might be to only be having the best habits but this is a process and takes us time to get there.

Still don't believe me? Results talk for themselves. Next time you are around unfit people *listen* to how they talk. They are constantly trying to 'give up' something whether it be sugar or fats or alcohol and then are in a cycle of guilt for not being able to give those things up completely.

However, if you look at a fit person they have good habits most of the time and whenever you are out with them it *seems* like they can just eat as much as they want without getting fat. It's because the fit people have good habits 80-90% of the time, so when they do want to indulge they have a bit of freedom to do so because they know their next meal will go straight back to their normal healthy choices. Whereas the unfit person is scared that they might spiral out of control. This is because they do not have the healthy habits to begin with!

Action Steps

1. Replace Bad Habits with better ones! E.g.

- Swapping a cappuccino every morning for an almond flat white

- Changing from Coke to Coke Zero

- Get off train 1 stop earlier on way home to hit 10,000 steps instead of 6,000

- Slowly increase weight on squats by 2.5kg every 2-4 weeks

2. Practice the healthy habit swaps CONSIS-TENTLY! Remember, what's simple to do is also simple to not do!

12. MIND-SET.

It's a fact that what your body does is controlled by your mind. So anytime you want your body to do something challenging you need to get your mind-set to work for you not against you. This is a big chapter so I'm gonna break it down into sub-sections.

12.1 You focus on the Negatives!

Most unfit people have a mind-set that sets them up for failure:

They focus on the negatives such as:

- Telling themselves training is not fun

- Or eating a healthy diet has to be boring

This overshadows all the positives and kills their willpower to even begin!

We must ask ourselves:

- What is the point of such a mind-set?

- Does it make it easier or harder to achieve results with this mind-set?

If we answer these questions honestly, it's clear that this mind-set does nothing to steer us in the direction of our goals. It just puts us off instead!

So what should we be doing instead?

Ask ourselves empowering questions! This now gives you the opportunity to answer in a productive way.

Such as:

How can I make my training as enjoyable as possible?

- A: I really like lifting weights and my goal is fat loss but I don't like running. But my trainer told me if I do supersets I can burn fat. Great I'll do that.

How can I make my healthy food super enjoyable for me?

- A: I love big salads with a variety of ingredients so I'm gonna do a big shop tonight and get all the ingredients I like that are healthy and make a bomb of a salad to last me for the next 2 days!

Or A: I love biscuits and ice cream; my trainer has written a blog on healthy desserts so I'm gonna use these ideas to make a nice dessert tonight.

By asking questions in this way, it allows our brains look for ways to resolve our problem rather than keep us IN the problem!

Action Steps

1. Write down 3 common negative phrases you tell yourself to do with fitness or health?

2. Using the examples above, write down an alternative way to say the question so it becomes an empowering question instead?

3. Write down the answers to each of these questions.

Unfit people:

- Experience a 'temporary' defeat such as not losing weight after 3 weeks of trying a new eating/training regime or current exercise routine is not working. So, they get disheartened and quit!

- The sad thing about this is that they will quit, gain more weight and go through an unhappy phase for a few months or years but then will ALWAYS decide to try again at some point. If only they had just persisted the first time, imagine where they would be now?

As I always tell my clients…*sometimes it can be a slow process but quitting won't get you there faster!*

Fit people:

Also have these same failures AND they also feel disheartened in the moment too.

- The fundamental difference is that fit people don't quit! They know that failure will happen again and again on their journey and it's just the way things go!

- They always ask themselves **empowering questions** which gives them the opportunity to learn and grow.

Examples of empowering questions include:

- What have I learned from this failure?

- What can I do better?

- How can I improve and not let this happen again?

There is a common theme with these questions; they all offer you the opportunity to get better.

1. Write down 2 situations where you failed in the past and then gave up.

2. For each situation write down an empowering question you could have told yourself to help steer you back on track.

3. Write down the answer to these empowering questions.

4. The next time you fail. Use an empowering question to get yourself out of the negative state and give yourself a chance to grow.

5. Remember, no matter what you mustn't quit! You just need to learn and adapt.

Hands up if you're a perfectionist. Keep your hands raised if either of these next two phrases resonate with you:

"If I can't do it perfectly, then I really don't want to do it at all."

"I will not begin an exercise routine unless I can do 5 days per week of training + be 100% perfect diet wise; because there's no point otherwise"

Now, do you think being a perfectionist is a good thing or a bad thing?

Socially, being a perfectionist is seen as a positive trait and as a result a lot of us like to be this way. However, most of us really have no idea the harm this outlook can have on us.

Have you ever put something off because you want it to be absolutely **100% perfect**?

Often we won't attempt many great things in life simply because we're scared that our efforts will turn out to be **less than perfect**, maybe even mediocre or worse – we fail entirely. So we don't try it at all.

And when you're looking at accomplishing something such as losing 20kgs of fat or trying to completely embody a healthy new lifestyle, you keep focusing on **how big** it is and don't begin because you don't feel comfortable breaking it down into small steps because you must do it **All**.

Unfit people often have this mentality so they end up:

- Not exercising AT ALL because they cannot commit to doing 1 hour per day 3 x per week.

- Or they think it's pointless eating well only some of the time, so they just eat badly until they are ready to commit to eating clean 100% of the time.

Fit people:

- Understand that they cannot be perfect in every way and certainly not all the time. Instead they focus their efforts on doing WHATEVER they can, whenever possible, no matter how little or inconsequential it may seem.

  - o So, if they can't make a full workout they go in and do 20 minutes at least.

  - o Or if they have a mega hectic week at work they do 1 session instead of the 3 they normally do.

  - o Or they're at a family dinner in an unhealthy restaurant. They choose the healthiest food possible on that menu.

- They know that something is ALWAYS better than nothing. And it is precisely this, that makes them successful in the long run!

- They break things down into small blocks until they are ready to commit to more e.g. they say 'okay I will start with going to the gym 1x per week. I may not lose any weight but I know it's the direction I should be going so I will start with that first'. Then as time goes on and they enjoy it they start finding ways to make time for another session.

Action Steps

1. Write down an example of where you have had an 'all or nothing' approach with fitness? And where would you be now if you had just began back then with a few small steps in the right direction?

2. Next time, why not try **taking action immediately** and instead of expecting perfect, allow yourself the room to make improvements over time. Begin in **bite-size steps** so you won't feel too overwhelmed to get started!

Remember that in almost 100% of cases, if you try something and mess it up you will be able to go back and try again until it's better.

13. TOO MUCH GUILT & MORALITY TOWARDS FOOD!

Nowadays with powerful food/cult groups (paleo, vegan, keto, IIFYM), as well as a huge influence from mainstream media/advertising/social pressures, people have now developed this unhealthy condition where they place huge moral and emotional views on food. (For the record I'm not talking about vegan's view on not eating meat).

Some common examples of good/bad food labelling include:

- 'All sugar is bad'

- 'Fat is bad because it makes you fat'

- If someone wants to eat chocolate or a dessert, deep down they feel they are committing some huge sin.

- 'Oh it's okay to eat as much avocado as you want because it's a good fat.'

- 'Carbs make you fat'

- 'Bread makes you fat'

- Or being proud to say things like 'Oh I only eat sweet potatoes but never normal potatoes'

Such labeling leads many people to having a really unhealthy relationship with food. And the worst thing is 'most' of these people literally have no idea what they are talking about. They completely misunderstand in what context the previous statements may hold any truth.

Another thing is laboling foods that are actually good, such as potatoes, as bad because they think only sweet potatoes are healthy, since they are what all the magazines are raving on about. I have met people who were genuinely so scared to eat a potato, being a 'carb', they believed they would instantly put on fat from one bite. True Stories.

The following should not be forgotten:

- We are an advanced species living on this planet that simply has adapted in such a way that we can use many foods as fuel for our bodies. This is mainly because we have many ways of cooking and preparing food which allows us to digest food that we would not otherwise be able to.

In my opinion, food is definitely something that can and should be enjoyed but it's also important to recognise that ultimately it is fuel for our body. Placing morals of good and bad on food does more harm than good, and can create a really unhealthy relationship with food. Of course it's important to know how each food affects us and this is why you have to be very careful about where you get your information from and who you listen to. Make sure they are a professional that clearly demonstrates and embodies an understanding of food for themselves and their clients.

Action Steps

1. Write down 3 situations when you have had a strong moral view towards food.

2. Upon reflection was your view real or taken out of context/exaggerated?

3. Do you think having this view has served you well or made you limit your food choices unnecessarily?

FYI: I am writing a nutrition manual which gives the full low down on nutrition fundamentals, best strategies to implement and best of all myth busting all the rubbish that is out there which confuses the hell out of normal people.

14. TRAPPED IN COMPLEXITY, WHEN THINGS COULD BE SO SIMPLE.

A lot of people don't realise that the things that we need to change in order for health to emerge are simple things.

Unfit people tend to overcomplicate things and create obstacles when there are none; making EVERY step in the direction of health seem an enormous burden to overcome! This is particularly common with the attention to detail/technical personality types.

Some examples of these unnecessary complications include:

- Going to a restaurant and immediately telling yourself that '**it's so hard/complicated to eat something healthy while eating out**' and therefore your health (diet) is a write off!

That's absolute rubbish! I guarantee you I could go to eat in any place and without much complication at all, still eat reasonably well.

- Getting so hung up on **what time** you 'should be' eating your foods or trying to use advanced methods such as carb cycling or variations of intermittent fasting, while the foundations (food choice and quantity) are all over the place.

Logically thinking about it, if I'm eating 600 calories more per day than my body needs, I will gain fat. It doesn't matter what time I'm eating if I'm simply eating too much.

- Focusing on every single rep **being so perfect** that you end up doing 10 reps of 1 exercise in a whole 1 hour workout! You get so caught up trying to get perfect form that you **don't work at the intensity** you are supposed to so never achieve anything.

I'm all about good technique but there is a limit on obsessive behavior.

Break it down to simplicity!

The most important thing is the fundamentals of your goal!

If your goal is to drop body fat, then you need to do the following:

- Eat enough quality protein and green veg.

- Burn more than you are eating! AND do it consistently over time.

- Make your workouts have only 60-90 secs rest between each exercise so you keep the heart rate high enough to burn fat.

- That is it! Don't over complicate.

Action Steps

1. Write down 3 situations where you have made something relatively simple, way more complicated than it needs to be?

2. What simple things can you do, starting from tomorrow, that will get you closer in the direction of your goals?

15. WILLPOWER vs ENVIRONMENT: WHO WINS?

Unfit people have this idea in their head that the reason they are not where they want to be is because they 'do not have enough willpower' or they don't have the same amount as successful people do. While there is a small amount of truth in that, I'm here to tell you that relying on willpower is BS! The smart people understand that as humans we are all flawed and so they use their environment to help get the best out of them instead of relying solely on willpower.

Here are some of the things the willpower gang tell themselves:

- 'I must have more willpower'

- 'I must be more motivated'

- 'No its okay if everyone around me eats chocolates I will just use my willpower to resist all temptation'

How realistic is it that they will do the above day in day out? The unfit guys seem to think it's doable.

The reality looks something more like the following:

Wake up, head to work. You get your coffee and skip the croissant because you're being 'healthy' and making up for a heavy night before. Then at lunch you go for a salad because once again you are being 'healthy'. You spend the whole afternoon saying no to little biscuits and stuff that your colleagues keep offering you. Then you finally get home. Your brain is fried and you are knackered. There is no food in your fridge and you are craving food and your partner fancies pizza. You can't say no anymore cos you're fed up! So you have the pizza and you've gone past the point where you feel bad about what you've had. You fancy something sweet and you open your drawers and all you have is chocolates and sweets. You wake up the next day feeling guilty about what happened last night but also determined to attack the day with more willpower! ...the cycle continues.

The environment gang recognizes the limitation of relying on willpower ALL THE TIME so they do the following:

- Make sure their home is full of good ingredients and also has some tasty/healthy snacks for when their sweet tooth kicks in...because they know it will.

- They make sure their office desk, cupboard and fridge are also filled with the good stuff.

- Their partner is aware of their goals and also interested in training too so they help support each other, especially during dinners.

- If they are meeting a mate for dinner that they know they always end up drinking and eating loads with. They just make sure they eat less (only protein and veg) during that day so the total daily damage isn't as much.

Who do you think is the more successful of the two? Environment or Willpower gang?

Get your environment working for you!

1. What food you have in the house?

- Fill your fridge with fresh vegetables and lean cuts of meat (marinated)

- Fill your freezer with:

    ☐ Low calorie Frozen Pizzas

    ☐ Frozen Berries/ Grapes

    ☐ Oppo Ice Cream

- Fill your dessert cupboards with healthier snacks such as:

    ☐ Kallo Salt & Vinegar Rice Cakes

    ☐ Nairn's biscuits

    ☐ Fibre one Chocolate Brownies

SO when you do get home it's these items you will be tempted by which are much lower in calories, sugar & fat than the things you may currently have in your house. So even if you do go on a crazy binge; you will literally be doing 50% less damage!

2. Your Partner

I don't think people realize how much of an impact their partner has on their goals in general; but especially fat loss because of their influence on food.

- Tell them your goals and ask for their support. It's much easier if they are also health conscious too otherwise when you are trying to clear out the junk from your cupboards they will not be happy and a huge conflict may occur!

- Try to go to the gym together. It can be another way for you guys to bond while also achieving your fitness goals.

3. Your Friends

Okay so we all know that our friends can influence us. But some trainers tell their clients to just get new friends which always cracks me up because who is really gonna do that? My suggestion is not to change friends but adapt to how you hang with them.

You know they're a big drinker

- Cool, meet with them but drink lower calorie drinks such as gin and slim line tonic or go for straight whisky on the rocks.

You know they're a big eater

- Cool, just eat veggies and protein that day, that way you are satisfying nutritional requirements and eating less calories. So when you do meet them for food you will not be having a heavy meal plus loads of other stuff you have already eaten that day!

4. Meet new people at the gym/in classes.

- They are likely to be interested in health like you so you guys can hang out and support each other.

Action Steps

1. List 3 examples when you have over relied on willpower and it's not worked out well for you in the end.

2. Write down 3 ways you can get your environment working for you.

16. TRYING TO DO IT ALL ALONE!

At best you run the risk of having **slow progress.**

- You may go for an endless cycle of trial and error, taking years to improve and still may never be satisfied with results.

- There is a lot of conflicting info on the internet/social media, but it takes knowledge and expertise in that area to decipher the BS from the good stuff. Also most articles are written to help the masses so how do you know if that article can truly apply to you?

In the worst case you run the risk of **hurting yourself** from doing exercises incorrectly.

The fastest way to get results is hiring a coach that has got themselves and others where it is that you want to be; use and leverage their experience.

How do I know if they are good?

- Ask them for **examples of their work**; clients that have achieved the results you want.

Are they expensive?

- **Sure, if they are genuinely good at what they do** their most premium 1-2-1 service might initially appear to be a lot BUT if you compare it against the amount of money you could be wasting with a bad trainer where you still pay a moderate amount but learn nothing and get no results. Then sometimes paying more is better.

- Also, **monthly coaching** is a great option nowadays. You could be paying as little as **£150-200** per month for someone to take care of your nutrition, exercise routine, keep you accountable and do regular check-ups with you.

Do this for about 6 months and you could potentially have made one of the best investments in your health ever! You will know how to eat, how to train and have the habits of a fitter and healthier person. This can never be taken away from you.

Action Steps

1. Hire a Coach!

2. Contact me via my website www.fittestyou.co.uk

3. Otherwise, check who on social media is doing what you like and see what options they have.

You would think it's so simple:

Pay Coach + Do As Coach Says = Get Results

Unfortunately, this doesn't always happen. So, here are a few tips for you the client to get the most out of your coach/trainer. Assuming that you have done your research to find a coach that has got people the results that you want, **here are my tips:**

The main reason you hire a coach for their expertise is so you can get results. But people forget that they should listen to what their coach tells them.

1. **Remember** that you have hired them for their expertise and experience which means that they know more than you in this area!

2. **Follow their system and process.** They know the fastest way for YOU to get the results you want so it's wise for you to follow their advice.

A good coach will read your level so will give you realistic targets to aim for. These targets are different for most people so do not compare yourself against what other friends/ people on the internet are doing as you do not know their full story.

3. **Communicate** with them to get the most from your coach
   - How you are feeling

   - What you notice working

   - What's hard for you outside the gym

   - Feel free to ask questions about why you're doing something

This gives your coach the opportunity to respond to you and tailor things even more to your needs.

- Don't just sit there like some passive person watching time go by without saying anything.

4. If you are the skeptical type, decide you will give them and their methods a proper chance for a reasonable time frame (e.g. 1-2 months). If you do give them this chance, then make sure you REALLY make effort to embody the process and not be a cynic. A great coach will be so confident in their ability that they may be willing to guarantee your results. So check this with them.

CONCLUSION

If you have just skimmed through this book, go back again and follow all the Action Steps!

If you have done the action steps, you will already be miles away from the old 'Unfit' mind-set you once lived in and now operating from a 'Fit' mind-set instead. If you continue to embody and apply all you have learned from the book, you will undoubtedly become the fittest version of yourself and no longer 'fail in fitness'.

If you feel that this book has really resonated with you and want to work with me directly, feel free to contact me via my website: www.fittestyou.co.uk Otherwise continue to enjoy all you have learned from the book.

To your success!

Alex

Printed in Great Britain
by Amazon